Printed By Createspace, An Amazon.com Company

Made in United States
Troutdale, OR
02/09/2025

28781083R00075